❧ Beauty ❧
❧ Inside Out ❧

80 Ways to Become
Positively Unforgettable

Kare Anderson
and
Kay Casperson

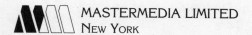

MASTERMEDIA LIMITED
New York

ISBN 1-57101-064-5
Library of Congress Catalog Card Number: 96-75776

Cover designed by David Charlsen
Text pages designed by Michael Woyton
Manufactured in the United States of America
10 9 8 7 6 5 4 3 2 1

BEAUTIFUL LEGACY OF LIVING

Recognize Your Most Unforgettable Snapshot

The power to define is the power to choose.

Were I to ask your friends to close their eyes, and let their minds go peacefully blank, and then I asked each of them to describe the first image that came to mind when I said someone's name, and then I said your name, what is the first image they would picture?

Would it be beautiful? Would it be all that you'd want it to be?

What is the lasting image that you want to leave behind you after every interaction in your life?

———◦○◦———

TIP: Love each moment of being alive and you will be more alive.

BEAUTIFUL VISION
Know What You Stand For

Opportunity is often inconvenient.

When you hold onto a vision of a higher purpose in life, you create a larger-than-life image that people want to share. Your sense of purpose:

★ fuels your energy and passion;
★ gives you clarity and concentration;
★ reduces stress because you make choices more easily;
★ attracts people by its beauty.

Your vision keeps you—and others around you—on a more fulfilling life journey because you notice the clouds in the sky more than the rocks in your path. Nourish that vision inside (in your mind and heart) and out (with your body) so that it grows in beauty. Make your daily actions reflect what you stand for.

———◦◦◦◦———

TIP: Make every action a reflection of your higher vision of yourself and of others.

BEAUTIFUL GOODNESS

Respond to the Longing for Love

*Power resides not in aggressiveness,
but in conscious choice.*

Life's sweetest moments take place when we are bathed in the love of others. Our most universal longing is for more love in our lives.

Our parents trained us to seek love and approval by being "good" in one of three ways: being good at doing (our accomplishments or leadership), being good to others (helping, putting others first) and/or being good-looking (concerned about physical appearance).

Being good in those ways are all attempts to draw more attention to ourselves. None is as successful as a fourth way of being good: by making others feel good when they are around you.

Focus the spotlight on them and they will shine and love you for the experience. Support the beauty in others, and others will bring out yours.

———◦◦◦———

TIP: Leave a memorable afterimage of yourself by focusing the camera of attention on others.

BEAUTIFUL PONDS
Create Breathtaking Reflections

Strengths spread just as fears do.

When others feel good about themselves when they are around you, they'll:

★ "see" the qualities in you that they most cherish, some of which you may not even have;

★ go out of their way to support you;

★ praise and care for you.

When they don't like the way they are when they are around you, they'll:

★ blame you for it;

★ "see" qualities in you they don't like in other people;

★ deny you credit for your accomplishments;

★ shut you out.

Your every word, move, sound and look make people feel better or worse. No action is neutral.

Do you dwell on others' mistakes or on their "magic moments"?

Do others become more upbeat or downcast around you?

———⋙∘✦∘⋘———

TIP: Whatever you praise, you'll cause to flower.

BEAUTIFUL MIND-SET SWITCH
Make Irritating People into Unlikely Allies

Resenting others is a way of never leaving them.

Your biggest opportunity to grow more beautiful is through the person who most upsets you. Contact with that person forces you to face your "hot buttons," enabling you to learn how to choose to act, rather than spontaneously reacting. If that person leaves your life before you've learned your lesson, someone else will arrive to play the same role.

People who rub you the wrong way have been trained by their parents to be good at what you're not good at. Watch them to learn how to practice their kind of "being good"—your underdeveloped other side. These "antagonists" can even become your allies. Talk with them about your different talents. Forge agreements to support each other. You'll still bump heads, but you'll know why.

———◦∞◦———

TIP: Don't let somebody else determine your behavior.

BEAUTIFUL OPPORTUNITY
Choose to Live Your Beauty

The sweetest revenge is a well-lived life.

When you point out to someone that he or she is behaving like a jerk, the person will go out of his or her way to prove it to you further. Tensions rise. Options fall.

When you start getting upset, reliving such incidents, those hot feelings can consume you. Instead, once you know your feelings, move to making a choice. You can:

★ change how you are acting (the only behavior over which you have control);

★ accept the situation and give it no more energy, turning your attention elsewhere;

★ remove yourself from the situation, whether it is a room, a job or a relationship.

You are more agitated, powerless and unattractive before you've made a choice than after. After you've made a choice, you become more positively powerful.

TIP: When others are being difficult, praise parts of them you do like.

BEAUTIFUL EASE
Read Your Body and Return to Innocence

Stress is often caused not by an event itself,
but by our responses to the event.

Children toddle, their innocence showing in the looseness of their bodies. Until children experience fear, they don't hold tight reactions to it in their bodies. We adults have tightened our muscles around every major experience of pain and anger. And others harden up instinctively in reaction to our moments of tightness.

Your body speaks to you all the time, telling you what your own needs are. It is your best living record of your life. How you respond to it is advertised in how you hold your body.

Take a personal body examination. Where do you hold your tension: your neck, shoulders, tummy or jaw? Are you shouldering the world's responsibilities, or perpetually drooping? In your determined drive toward success, do you plant your feet solidly on the ground in hostility and defiance? Do you have a forward-leaning posture of taking control?

TIP: Listen to your body. It's the best early warning system of what you are feeling.

BEAUTIFUL SIGNATURE STYLE
Let Your Body Speak Well for You

Whenever you throw mud, you get dirty.

When you instinctively tense up in anticipation of a hostile action from someone, you increase the chances of getting that action. Your heartbeat goes up, your skin temperature down. Others tense their bodies in reaction to yours. Their bodies mimic yours. Tense bodies get misaligned, use more energy, look less powerful. The more frequently you tense up, the longer your body stays tense. Eventually muscle tension becomes permanent. You even lose the awareness of being tense.

Women are more likely to shut down, be still, drain energy. Men are more likely to act out, move more, use up energy.

Loosen your body's reactions and others soften toward you. Regain the fluid innocence of childhood by:

★ exercising;
★ getting a massage or other body work;
★ giving love.

Exercise regularly to stay limber so you'll move gracefully through life.

TIP: Change how you hold your body and you'll change how you hold your emotions.

BEAUTIFUL BELIEF
Move Toward Happiness

There are two kinds of pain: pain of risk and pain of regret.

You can act your way into feeling better. Why? Because there is no such thing as "acting." When you act out one of the universally expressed emotions—anger, love, hurt, disgust, sadness—your body reacts as if the emotions were "real."

Just as a garden hose has a "memory"—when you wind it up it curls naturally in one circular direction, and resists all others—your body has a habitual response it moves into for each basic emotion.

Whatever emotion you choose to physically act out becomes your primary feeling of the moment. Notice and remember your body movement and posture when you feel happy. Next time you start feeling a negative emotion such as anger, move from thinking about that feeling to physically acting out the "happy feeling" posture and motions you've memorized. Move your body into acting happy and your heart and mind can follow.

———◦◦◦———

TIP: It is easier to act your way into a better way of feeling than to feel your way into a better way of acting.

Make Every Move Count

***The only difference between a slap
and a caress is the speed of the motion.***

Slow down and what you are chasing will come around and catch you. Maintain an economy of body in the beginning of a situation and when you want to appear credible.

For women especially, physical understatement conveys assurance, power, an air of grace. When women with less frequent, fewer, lower and slower movements do move, their motions have considerably more credibility and dramatic impact. The average female American executive makes approximately eighty different movements from the time she enters a meeting room until she is settled. The average male executive goes through thirty motions.

Extra motion is a denial of your personal power, an avoidance of direct contact with others, a "busyness" that belies your central beauty. Like a superb tennis player, aim for no extra motions. Your overall game is dramatic to watch.

———————⊰⊱———————

TIP: Go on a body-motion reduction diet.

BEAUTIFUL GESTURES
Less Is Often More

Your face often reveals how you feel, and your body movements show the intensity of your feelings.

A woman reveals her intensity through her "hand dance"—inadvertently expressing her feelings through rapid, frequent gestures. Men tend to "leak" their intense feelings through their feet. Sitting with crossed legs, a man may keep his body still while twitching his raised foot.

As well, when one of two groups of men and women was instructed to smile and gesture more frequently than was the other group, those group members were described as more friendly than the others. Yet the women who gestured most were viewed as more shallow and less thoughtful than the women who gestured less frequently.

Gestures can trivialize an interaction. Used sparingly they add interest. Use fewer, lower and slower gestures to look beautifully self-confident.

———◦◦◦◦———

TIP: The person who moves the most appears to have the least to say.

BEAUTIFUL BEGINNINGS
Bring People Together in Body and Spirit

Like streams joining a river, communities grow stronger when people flow together.

Ceremonies create unity. For example, in certain churches the pastor asks people to greet others around them. Afterward everyone feels closer. Why? Three things got them in sync:

★ They've safely touched (shaking hands or lightly touching the top of someone's hand is a nonthreatening physical contact).

★ They've smiled warmly at each other.

★ They've turned the trunks of their bodies as they moved to face those behind them.

When people are in sync with each other, they feel safer and more connected. As your rapport builds, people imitate each other's body motions. Your motions begin to flow together like an unfolding ballet. Two people who are deeply in love often appear to flow in one motion.

───────◈◦◈◦◈───────

TIP: Strengths spread just as fears do.

BEAUTIFUL BONDING
Support Others' Positive Passions

You could be the only angel in another's life.

People give you their "operating manual," telling you what makes them run smoothly when they describe someone they like or dislike. When you want others' support, your first instinct is to discuss what is important to you (self-centered) or to give background information (boring). Instead, display and refer to the qualities others most like.

First address others' current pressing interest or self-image. "Ride the energy" of their strongest emotions and you'll gain their support with less effort.

Describe how your request supports their most passionate beliefs about themselves and the world. Relate your ideas to what they most value. For example, someone who believes in detailed thinking will like a plan that you characterize as being well thought out. A person who likes adventures will be most interested in an outing you describe as a new experience.

TIP: If you want others' trust and support, address their interests first and frequently.

BEAUTIFUL WORD PICTURES
Say the Unforgettable

Whoever most vividly characterizes a situation usually determines how others see it, discuss it and act upon it.

Give people just facts and they may argue or forget. Give them a vivid word picture and leave an indelible memory. There are four secrets to speaking unforgettably:

★ Relate what you say to the three core life experiences: family, work and home.

★ Refer first to others' current interests then to your own.

★ Since motion increases memory, involve others in motion as you speak, such as by walking together or shaking hands.

★ Be specific, provide vivid details, and avoid general conclusions. Say "It's cobalt blue and crimson red" not "It's colorful."

People will remember what you say and associate your beautiful words with you as they see you saying them.

———◦◦◦◦———

TIP: Speak in vivid word pictures and others will forever remember what they saw you say.

BEAUTIFUL FIRST IMPRESSION

Act Right

We do not see things as they are. We see them as we are.

First impressions are formed within seven to twenty seconds—and require significant events to change.

Women and men form first impressions differently. Most men must first find others credible in order to form a positive opinion of them. Likability is secondary.

For women, the reverse is usually true. Women must instinctively like others first, then find them credible. A woman who doesn't like her boss is much more likely to let the boss see that that feeling than a man would be. The lessons?

- ★ When meeting a man for the first time, bring out your most credible side.
- ★ When meeting a woman for the first time, bring out your most likable side.
- ★ Men want to feel respected and competent.
- ★ Women want to feel cherished and noticed.

———◦◦◦◦———

TIP: Connect with others through what they most value.

BEAUTIFUL GAZE

Stare to Care

Only the unintelligent get bored.

Focus on the person with whom you are talking as if no one else exists at that moment. The person will bask in that rare act of respect. Others are attracted to attentiveness, even when it is not directed at them.

The face is the most memorable part of the body, the eyes are the most memorable part of the face. Eyes can project confidence and inspire trust. Make yours say, "I am listening," reinforcing the warmth and interest in your tone. Use your eyes as a steadying force, a credibility builder. Initiate a gaze. Hold it for a natural period of time.

Don't dilute your power by casting your eyes down or letting them dart away. People desire eye contact, even if they don't give it.

Don't assume that others are not paying attention even if they are looking away. They may be shy, thinking about what you are saying or reflecting a cultural difference. Don't try to make them look you in the eye.

———◦∞◦———

TIP: Your receptive gaze is your visible sign of respect.

BEAUTIFUL VISION

Help Them Like What They See So They'll Listen

Failure is no more fatal than success is permanent.

People see before they hear. Our brains receive what we see at 186,000 miles per second, the speed of light, and process what we hear more slowly, at only 750 miles per hour.

That is why people's minds can wander, even as you say, "Hello, let me introduce myself. My name is.... Who are you?" They are processing what they are seeing, not what they are hearing. They are much more likely to remember your face than your name.

If others do not like or trust what they see in you they will discount what you say, even if your message is true and/or conveys information they need.

Put your attention to how you appear to your listeners before attempting to get them to listen to you.

———

TIP: Say what you want others to hear only after they have seen what they need to see.

BEAUTIFUL REVEALING

See Both Sides of Others in Their Faces

Look to others' positive intent, especially when they appear to have none, not for them, but for yourself.

We are all, literally, two-faced, because the vertical halves of our faces are affected by discrete nerve systems on opposite sides of the brain. The left side is more likely to show negative emotions, the right reveals the positive personality. The left side reflects basic life attitude. The "social mask" of controlled responses appears on the right.

The right brain, through the left eye, is more actively involved in observing the world. When you face someone, your left eye is across from the other person's right side. You are more aware of the other's right side, which is connected with the left or "logical" side of the brain. You are not facing the half that most reveals underlying feelings.

Tɪᴘ: Look to the left side of others' faces to see their logical side and to the right to glimpse their underlying emotions.

BEAUTIFUL INSIGHT
See Your Life Patterns

*The opposite of a fact is a falsehood, but
the opposite of one profound truth may
very well be another profound truth.*

Get out old and recent group photos of family and friends to see your relationship patterns. Who is standing next to whom? Who appears at the center? Who's pretending to fight? Who's standing close? Who's hugging whom or standing away? Whose body is directed at another's? Whose body is enclosing someone else's? Whose is covering up someone else's? Who do you seem to lean into, stand by? Who wanted to be close or far from you? How do the people in your life now replicate the same patterns? Do you have a spouse who acts the same way as your parent of the same sex?

Look at recent group photos for similar themes. If you are looking at pictures of the same group over time, notice that there are seldom radical changes, only gradations of the power balance as we age.

———⟨∘⊙∘⟩———

TIP: Look at your group photos over time to see the patterns of your relationships.

BEAUTIFUL BALANCE
Speak So Others Want to Help

*Adversity can yield richer
learning experiences than joy.*

We react sooner, quicker, longer and stronger to negative incidents than to positive ones. We use more intense, colorful language to characterize the negative parts of a story, and are more concise describing the positive.

When you have potentially troubling news to share, keep the listener's attention by reporting it without emotion-laden words. Praise the positive. Describe the negative in factual, nonjudgmental language and the positive in vivid emotional words. You will come across as reasonable and preserve the relationship.

———◦◦◦◦———

TIP: Get your complaint noticed and keep your image clean. Report the negative news simply and generously praise the positive.

BEAUTIFUL ANGLES
Lean Toward Power

*Beliefs shape our experiences
more than experiences shape our beliefs.*

Because of their childhood training, women tend to sit and stand in public primly straight with their hands in their laps or their arms and legs together in power-robbing, symmetrical body poses that make them look—and act—passive.

But when we sit comfortably and slightly asymmetrically, we look more at ease and more powerful, without losing femininity. For example, suppose you rest one arm lightly across the back of the adjacent chair. You'll look more assured and interesting. When you stand, position one arm slightly differently than the other, and you'll appear more powerful. If, however, you choose an extremely asymmetrical stance, such as leaning sharply against a counter, you'll look sloppy or disrespectful.

Pick slightly asymmetrical poses that are you. Use them when you most need to feel and look confident.

———◦◦◦———

TIP: Become more credible with slightly asymmetrical body poses.

◄ 22 ► BEAUTIFUL BODY SPACIOUSNESS
Expand Your Territory to Extend Your Power

What you do not say often says it all.

One's sense of power is unconsciously projected in how much space one takes up. In our culture, men tend to take up more space and to insert themselves into others' personal space more than do women. By taking up less space, women look more passive and shrink their power.

Let your body take up more space and appear more powerful. Place one arm over an empty chair to extend your turf and power, especially if you are short, nonwhite or female. Take up too much space and people will resent and resist you. When a woman takes up too much space, such as leaning back with both arms around adjacent, empty chairs, men tighten in disapproval. When a woman holds her arms and legs close together, she tends to get overlooked, interrupted.

Take early action:

- ★ Place a briefcase near you to expand your turf.
- ★ Lean forward at the table with your elbows extended.
- ★ Make some wide gestures when speaking.

TIP: Take up more space and you'll also get more attention.

BEAUTIFUL COLORS OF SOUND
Hear Others Out

Our emotions fuel our energy.

Want to know how strongly someone feels? People reveal far more by their tones than their words.

Ignore their words for a moment. Instead notice telltale signs such as voice pitch, which, for seventy percent of Americans, goes up when feelings get more intense. Breathing, voice tightness, speed and level change. In fear, people often speak more slowly, in sadness, at a lower pitch. As you become attuned to others' sounds, you'll hear their emotions escalate before they say so in words.

Are the words you hear consistent with the speaker's depth of feeling? Check for congruency by noticing whether the sound of the speaker's voice is giving the same message as his or her body and words.

Stay aware of your own feelings by tuning into your voice.

———◦◦◦———

TIP: Listen for truth in the sound of someone's voice.

BEAUTIFUL MUSIC
Let Your Voluptuous Voice Envelop

Shut people out and they shut up.
Bring people in and they open up.

Too often people speak as if time is short. We bluntly crush words together as if we were forcing them into a trash compactor. A rat-a-tat-tat machine gun speaking style may spew more information, but it also blasts others away, flattening memory and feelings.

The faster you speak the more you sacrifice the color, intensity and flow that pulls others toward you. When you talk too long, others feel ignored or subjugated. Speak in light sprints, if you must, rather than marathons. Make your words compelling in their brevity and low tone. Draw others in. Practice musical variety in your pacing. Add lushness to the tone and level of your voice. People lean in, entranced by the sound of a lilting voice.

TIP: Set a softer mood in a hardened world with a soft voice.

BEAUTIFUL SILENCE

Use Pauses to Preserve Precious Moments

Sip your drink reverently as if it is the axis on which the whole earth revolves, slowly, evenly, without rushing toward the future. Only this actual moment is life.

Gypsy Rose Lee said, "Anything worth doing well is worth doing slowly." The lack of movement or sound has peculiar power. A stillness or pause may be your most persuasive word. Leave gaps in which you and your words can be absorbed. You will also be demonstrating your desire for listeners' opinions.

Pause for five full seconds after you have made an important point. It will seem like a longer time to you than it will to your listeners, but you will have suspended time.

How do you feel when someone else is dominating the conversation? When you speak sparingly and use dramatic pauses, your appearance of ease gains you the control.

The most powerful messages are often those conveyed without words. Whoever speaks the most rarely has the most power.

———◦◦◦———

TIP: Give small silences in conversation as if sharing precious gifts.

BEAUTIFUL BRILLIANCE
Convey Color-Full Feelings

Demonstrate your feelings and intent with color.

Colors affect our perceptions and health because we all react to them. When we see red, our pulse and respiration quickens and our blood pressure goes up. Want to spark a relationship or make an impression at an important meeting? Use red.

Make your home feel like a sanctuary with dark blue for rest, contentment and security. Display dark green to convey feelings of stability, consistency and self-confidence. For an open, spirited discussion, fill an area with yellow, which supports feelings of optimism and open-mindedness. Cover a room with rainbow streamers for a celebration.

———◦◦◦———

TIP: Change your colors to change your moods. Change colors and scent and you'll feel different faster.

BEAUTIFUL SCENTS OF LIFE
Smell to Know Your Needs

Act as if the world is going to treat you well.

Smell is our most directly emotional sense and, thus, the fastest way to recognize our underlying feelings. (Women have a better sense of smell than men do.) More than any other sense, scent causes strong approach and avoidance emotional triggers.

To renew, refresh or romance, return to the use of scent. Scent helps form love bonds, yet if a woman doesn't like a man's smell, she won't like him. Scent your body and surroundings to evoke the right emotion:

> Peppermint as a reviver.
>
> Jasmine as an antidepressant.
>
> Mint and citrus for bursts of energy.
>
> Rose as a mood lifter.
>
> Lavender, honey and vanilla for comfort.
>
> Geranium for mood leveling.
>
> Rosemary as a booster.

Scent domino-sized pieces of paper and distribute them in your drawers, letters, car and bedroom.

———◦∞◦———

TIP: Scent to support your serenity or your sensuality.

BEAUTIFUL POWER

Respect the One Most Ignored

Life is the movie; death is just a photograph.

A famous basketball player once went to a celebrity charity tennis match. People immediately started walking toward him. He quickly surveyed the gathering, saw the charity's dedicated bookkeeper sitting by herself and strode up to her with outstretched arms before anyone could reach him.

Every group of people has a power pattern of relationships, like invisible threads, among them. People gain attention by the power they've acquired through:

- ★ position
- ★ money
- ★ star status celebrity

- ★ charisma
- ★ good looks
- ★ an inner beauty

When the person with the most threads of power directs attention to the person with the least, different combinations of people begin talking to each other in new ways. Conversations take unexpected turns. People see new sides of each other.

TIP: How you spend your time is how you show your values.

BEAUTIFUL RECONCILIATION
The Ten Minute Rule

"Love is not always power." That may be as good a description of the human predicament as we are likely to get.

If you are involved in an argument that seems unresolvable, consider that one of two things might have occurred:

By repeating your arguments several times, each of you has become more convinced of your own view and less open to hearing the other's.

If an argument lasts longer than ten minutes, you are probably not discussing the real point of disagreement. One or both of you may have an underlying grudge or hurt that is not being directly expressed in the surface argument. Until you can uncover the real point of contention and resolve it, or at least acknowledge that it exists, you won't get out of your "fighting" script.

———◦◦◦———

TIP: Whenever an argument lasts longer than ten minutes, the arguers are probably not arguing about the real conflict.

BEAUTIFUL SHARED EXPERIENCE

First Things First: Show Your Love

When underlying feelings hinder you,
look for other feelings.

This is one couple's promise to each other: Whenever they come into each other's company, they first exchange a kiss and a few words. Their first priority is to connect with each other.

When you awaken, when you go out and when you return, spend at least four minutes sharing a touch, a few words and a smile with your loved one. Even if you do not feel like being nice, do it anyway. Like the welding that forges a strong joint between two pipes, these moments strengthen your bond so that it doesn't crack during inevitable hard times.

This commitment is most important for the person in the relationship who is getting the most attention or feeling the most time pressed. Keep up the "insurance coverage" on your relationship by gratefully making the emotional payments it requires.

———◦◦◦◦———

TIP: Never stop demonstrating to the ones you love that you put them first.

BEAUTIFUL ATTENTION
Men: Ask So a Woman's Heart Can Open

You have to be present to win.

Six powerfully simple words, "Please tell me more about that," promote peacekeeping between the sexes. Any man can make any woman feel more respected or cherished by making that statement. Why?

Most women share a common desire for their relationships with the opposite sex: more apparent attentiveness. Women want to feel heard. When a man asks to hear more, and looks at a woman and leans toward her at the same time, the woman's heart is more likely to open to his.

This statement, which is also used by successful trial lawyers and therapists, is also useful when your mind is blank and you need to buy time and when you are spitting mad and need time to cool off.

———◦◦◦———

Tip: Give a woman the words she most needs to hear and you'll both feel closer.

BEAUTIFUL COUPLE
Deepen His Commitment to You

*As we set ourselves free from our own fears,
our presence liberates others.*

Encourage conversation about the feelings that you want to deepen. Saying something out loud makes it more real. When a man says something sweet to you, make him feel good. Ask him to elaborate and be supportive as he does. The more he speaks about his feelings, the more strongly he believes them. (Conversely, don't ask a man to elaborate on the things he doesn't like, or he will feel them more intensely, allowing them to cloud his positive feelings for you.)

The more actions one takes on behalf of an idea, the more intensely one believes it. For example, ask a customer what he likes best about your product, nod in approval as he responds and seek elaboration verbally and in writing, offering a gift for his input. The customer will be more committed to his views, more likely to tell others.

———◦○◦———

TIP: The more a man describes his warm feelings for you, the more deeply he believes them.

BEAUTIFUL STYLE
Unveil Your Personality

Let your personal style shine!

Your personality determines the style of clothing to which you'll be most attracted. If you're in the mood for fun or feeling playful, show it with color or whimsical pattern. When your wardrobe complements your outward energy, you become a complete picture of your personality.

———◦◦◦◦———

TIP: Do not be afraid of what other people may think. Be true to yourself to be beautiful.

BEAUTIFUL WRAPPING
Determine Your Look

*Your individual style should be inspired
by what most interests you.*

Use fashion magazines, style shows and catalogs as guides to determine what type of fashion look is most appealing to you. For example, are you most attracted to a romantic style (i.e. florals, flowing skirts, etc.), a fashion-forward style (hot colors and patterns, dramatic lines, etc.) or a classic style (subtle tones, traditional suits, etc.)? Make your own decisions about fashion based upon your own feelings.

TIP: Determine what you like and suit yourself. If you wear clothes that are not you, it shows!

BEAUTIFUL SEARCH
Shop Smart

Having style doesn't have to be expensive.

Just as good grooming and staying healthy are habits you learn, good shopping strategies can also be learned.

Just before your next shopping trip, take the time to carefully look at your existing wardrobe. When you're shopping, you'll be thinking about styles and colors that will complement the things that you already own, offering you savings and versatility. Sometimes buying one new skirt, jacket or pair of slacks will create several new outfits. Or adding a bright blouse will give an old suit new life.

———❈———

TIP: Take a fresh look at what's in your closet before your next shopping trip.

BEAUTIFUL PAUSE
Patience Pays

Allow yourself the luxury of time when creating your own style.

Think carefully about your image and don't compromise. Never shop on your lunch hour or in between appointments. Impulsive purchases often look impulsive. Most people will purchase an expensive jacket or blouse with far less consideration than purchasing a household appliance at the same cost. Your wardrobe is a serious investment, the only investment that you carry with you each day. Treat it with care, give it the time that it deserves and you will be rewarded with compliments.

Consider your "cost per wearing."

⊰∘◦∘⊱

TIP: Give your personal style the time that it deserves.

BEAUTIFUL STATURE
Stand Tall

*If you stand tall, you will exude a look
of confidence and control.*

The way that you carry yourself is very important. Try this simple exercise: In front of a mirror, stand comfortably in your normal posture. Take a good look at yourself. Next, stand as tall as you can, shoulders back, head held high. Tighten your abdominal muscles. Do you notice a difference? Most people do. Practice this exercise regularly. Your clothes will fall better on your body, and you'll notice a difference in how you look and how people perceive you.

TIP: Practice posture and build confidence.

BEAUTIFUL BOUQUET

Complementing Colors

*Make sure that what you're wearing conveys
the mood or message that you want others to notice.*

Colors play a very large role in how you look and feel. Never let your wardrobe control you. If you are getting compliments on your garment all day instead of on how great you look in it, the color of your outfit may be overpowering you.

———————

TIP: Never conflict, always complement with color.

BEAUTIFUL PURGE
Cleaning Out Clutter

You've taken the trip to style.
Now get rid of the baggage.

If you've followed the previous six tips, you've determined your "look," learned how to shop smart and chosen colors that work for you. Now it's time to come to terms with your closet. Anything that's not right for you does not belong in your wardrobe. If you haven't worn it for two seasons, it must go.

Once you've separated out the clutter, you can make a donation to a clothing bank or make a trip to a consignment shop. This is something that should be done every year, without exception. You'll find you'll look and feel better and more organized.

———◦◦◦———

TIP: If you don't use it, lose it.

BEAUTIFUL COORDINATION
Organization Is a Must!

The key to beautiful style is an organized closet.

Now that you've done the weeding, group your clothing by season and category. Keep fall and winter clothing together separate from spring and summer. If you have the space, you may even consider separate racks or closets. Jackets or blazers belong together. Casual attire should be separated from dressier outfits. This will make it easier to take stock when updating your wardrobe.

———◦◦◦◦———

TIP: An organized closet coordinates style!

BEAUTIFUL BASE
Feet First

Shoes are a terrific, often neglected, accessory.

Many of us have a tendency to own too many shoes or shoes that we never wear. To keep footwear in order, shoe racks are a must. And, just like clothes, shoes should be organized by season, style and color. Once you're organized, you'll quickly notice your needs. Too many black pumps, maybe?

TIP: Using shoe racks will save you time and money.

BEAUTIFUL BRAIN
The Mind Controls the Aging Process

Reprogram your mind and take control of how you age.

Never think or say things like, "I'm not getting any younger" or "I'm over the hill." Replace those negatives with positive thoughts and words such as "I feel great at any age" or "I'm not getting older, I just keep getting better every day!" A young attitude will keep you fresh.

———◦◦◦◦———

TIP: Think young to look young.

BEAUTIFUL ACTION
Do It Because It Feels Good

Working out makes you feel good!

Studies show that exercise is not only healthy but it is also an excellent mood elevator. Most people relate working out to slimmer hips, thinner thighs or tighter buns. But the important thing to remember is that working out makes you feel good! If you redirect your attention from a discipline approach to working out to how good you feel when you practice healthful habits, you'll have a healthier body and mind!

———◇◆◇———

TIP: Work out to feel good inside!

BEAUTIFUL LOCOMOTION
No More Excuses

A little stretch can go a long way!

For most of us, lack of time is the most popular excuse for not implementing a fitness program. What many don't realize is that physical fitness can be easily incorporated into our daily routines. Here are a few examples:

★ Take the stairs at least part of the way rather than waiting for the elevator.

★ Walk a bit and board the bus a couple of stops down the line.

★ If you drive to work, park ten minutes away and walk the rest of the distance.

★ Exercise the muscles in your buttocks by tightening them, holding the position for five seconds, relaxing them, then repeating while standing in line or sitting for long periods of time.

★ Do desk exercises such as twisting your torso slightly to each side and squeezing your abdominal muscles.

———⊸◦◦◦⊷———

TIP: Make time, not excuses, to become fit.

BEAUTIFUL NOISE
Exercise to Music

Keep the intensity of your workout, not the stress.

Music, according to research, affects physical responses. People can achieve the same intensity of work while exercising, but place less demand on the heart, when listening to music. Exercising to music can produce relaxation without sacrificing the benefits of the workout.

———❖———

TIP: Use music to motivate and relax.

BEAUTIFUL GLOW

Your Body Type Determines Your Workout

One type of exercise is not right for every body.

You can define your body with proper diet and exercise, but your shape is, to a certain degree, genetically determined. For example, a tall thin equally proportioned person who exercised regularly on a Stairmaster would be most likely to tone and tighten. A shorter, more shapely person would most likely add mass with the same exercise plan.

To successfully get the results you need, set a goal that works for your body shape. Ask a professional trainer to help you determine what exercises will best help you accomplish your goals.

———❈———

TIP: Let your physique and goals dictate your physical fitness program.

BEAUTIFUL GRAZING
Don't Be Afraid to Eat

You don't have to diet hard to have a beautiful body.

The reality is that the weight return rate is much higher after a diet, especially a crash diet. Learn how and what to eat instead of concerning yourself with how little you can eat. Eating smaller meals and regular healthy snacks will increase your metabolism and burn more fat than will eating one or two big meals a day.

———⊙⊙⊙⊙———

TIP: Smaller portions of healthy foods eaten more often will keep you trim.

BEAUTIFUL BEGINNING
The Right Start Is a Good Breakfast

*Breakfast is important to get the day
(and your metabolism) going.*

Here are pointers for a healthier start to your day:

★ Eat fruits first (you might then be too full for the peanut butter toast!).
★ Purchase low-fat pancakes and toast them instead of frying them.
★ Crisp frozen hash brown patties with cooking spray in a nonstick skillet.
★ Switch to Canadian bacon; it has half the fat of regular bacon.
★ Buy low-fat muffins; ordinary muffins can contain up to 12 grams of fat!
★ Lighten your coffee with evaporated skim milk.

———◦◦◦◦———

TIP: Fruit first to fill up.

BEAUTIFUL HALF-TIME

Healthy Lunches Energize Afternoons

At lunchtime, think healthy, not fat!

Try to prepare your lunch at home—you have many more options!

★ Substitute lemon juice and/or hot pepper sauce for mayonnaise when making tuna salad.

★ Use mustard instead of mayonnaise at all times!

★ Add as much lettuce and tomato as you'd like to salads and sandwiches.

★ To make a grilled cheese sandwich, toast the bread, put a slice of reduced-fat cheese between the slices and microwave.

★ Always use low-fat peanut butter. Or, buy natural peanut butter and pour off the oil that has risen to the top, which removes most of the fat.

———◆◆◆———

TIP: Add flavor and reduce fat.

BEAUTIFUL REWARD

Renewal with the Right Rewards

Give yourself sane self-indulgences.

Since having more time generally means eating more food, and since most of us have more time for dinner than any other meal of the day, eating smart at dinnertime is imperative.

- ★ When stir frying, add only a small amount of oil to vegetables. Augment their natural moisture by adding some water if needed.
- ★ Remember that white-meat chicken has approximately one-third less fat than dark meat. Pass on the skin!
- ★ Frying, from a nutritional standpoint, is the worst way to cook anything. Replace oils and batter with a nonstick spray.
- ★ Always buy lean meats.
- ★ When roasting meat, use a rack so the fat drips off. Grilled food is great!
- ★ Make low-fat oven fries instead of French fries by slicing baking potatoes into thin wedges, sprinkling them with low-calorie seasoning and roasting them in the oven.

───────◦◦◦◦◦───────

TIP: Think lean and limit oils.

BEAUTIFUL STRANDS
The Right Style for You

Having the hair style that is right for you is the first step to beautiful hair!

Choosing a hair style from a magazine or style book may not be a great idea since the person in the photo isn't you. Before choosing a style, ask yourself: "Does it suit my lifestyle, my face shape, the type of hair I have, my age? Is it a style that I could do myself at home?"

Don't be afraid to interview hair designers before giving one the very important job of creating and maintaining your personal look.

TIP: Consider your options before making a style change decision.

BEAUTIFUL BOTTLES
The Right Products

Finding the right hair style and stylist is one matter. Learning to properly care for your hair is another.

Choosing the right hair-care products is important, and it can be confusing. Always consider the color, type and condition of your hair before making a product decision. With so many products to choose from, you can surely find one that matches your overall needs. For example, choose a shampoo that cleanses as well as enhances color, or a daily conditioner that can also be used as a moisturizing treatment.

TIP: Don't compromise! Buy the products that are right for your hair.

BEAUTIFUL SHINE
Remove the Buildup

Hair fixatives such as gels, hair sprays and mousse cause buildup.

If you use these sorts of products on a daily basis, your hair will need a weekly deep cleaning to remove the buildup. Clarifying shampoos are designed to deep-clean the hair shaft and remove any buildup of fixatives to ensure healthy-looking hair. Otherwise, use a clarifying shampoo containing natural ingredients, instead of your daily shampoo, every other day. You'll improve the luster and overall condition of your hair.

———————

TIP: Use a clarifying shampoo on your hair on a regular basis.

BEAUTIFUL BREEZES
Be Careful About Drying

Blow-drying hair daily can be damaging.

The damage occurs when your hair is between the damp and dry stage. When you feel your hair start to become dry, switch to a cool setting on the blow-dryer. Stop before your hair is totally dry. Also, to minimize damage, deep condition your hair every other week by applying a natural moisturizing conditioner. Instead of rinsing it out immediately, towel wrap your hair for 15 to 20 minutes and then rinse.

———≼◦◦◦≽———

TIP: Never blow-dry your hair completely.

BEAUTIFUL VOLUME
Care for Your Hair Texture

In order to create beautiful hair styles, you must have products that compliment your hair texture.

Because there are many different hair types and textures, there are many styling products to choose from. Follow the suggestion that applies to your hair type:

★ **fine hair:** If you want to create more volume, use hair sprays, gels and mousse. Try to avoid shiners, silicone or other products that might build up on your hair. Stay away from products that tend to make hair look greasy.

★ **thick hair:** Use styling aids that are relatively light and come in liquid form; they comb through your hair easily. Shine products can be used to create a soft, smooth look.

★ **curly hair** (natural or permed): Create bouncy beautiful curls with liquid stylers, light gels or pomades. Stay away from mousse or thick gels.

★ **straight hair:** Create body with mousse and gels and don't be afraid to add a little shine!

———◦◦◦◦———

TIP: Consider the texture of your hair when choosing styling products.

BEAUTIFUL BOUNTY
Savvy Savings!

Price doesn't necessarily equate with quality when it comes to hair care products.

Ingredients are more important than designer names. You needn't shop at high-priced salons or department stores to find quality products. Savvy consumers shop at grocery and drug stores for hair and skin care products. If you look closely at labels, you'll find products of the same or better quality for much better prices. And you can use coupons for extra savings.

TIP: Grocery and drug stores offer the best values on hair-care products.

BEAUTIFUL BRUSHES
Essential Tools

Use the right tool for the job.

For beautiful hair and great style there are certain tools necessary for creating certain looks. Here are a recommended few:

- ★ **paddle brush:** To give long, thick hair a sleek smooth look, blow it dry using a paddle brush and styling gel.
- ★ **round brush:** For shaping and turning ends up or under, blow hair dry with a round, vented brush.
- ★ **Velcro rollers:** For adding volume and body, use Velcro rollers (large ones for volume and body, small ones for curl) on almost-dry hair (start at the top of the head). When hair is dry, remove the rollers, and comb and shape hair with a wide-toothed comb. Spray with a finishing spray.

———◦◦◦◦———

TIP: The right hair care tools are essential to creating the right look.

BEAUTIFUL HUES
Be Vibrant!

Coloring your hair is a fabulous way to get the excitement you're looking for.

When you look in the mirror do you see hair that is vibrant and shiny or dull and lifeless? Would you like to be a redhead, a blonde or a brunette? Professional color can give you just what you want!

When choosing a color, make sure you match it with your skin tone. If your skin tone has a yellowish cast, you should choose a golden or other warm shade. If your skin has more pink tones, choose an ash or other cooler shade of the color you want. Consult an expert hair stylist who has experience with color.

———◦∞◦———

TIP: Consider color to add life to your hair.

BEAUTIFUL PROTECTION
Sad But True—Avoid the Sun

Keep your skin young by limiting exposure to the sun.

Exposure to the sun's rays has been proven to be the major cause of aging skin. The good news is that you can still be in the sun for certain amounts of time without the damaging effects if you use a sunblock of at least SPF 15. Wearing a hat and sunglasses gives extra protection. If you live or travel to a place that has outdoor winter sports, sun protection is equally important, since the reflection from the sun on snow can be intense.

TIP: Wear a sunblock, rain or shine.

BEAUTIFUL SURFACE
Your Face Reflects What You Eat

We wear what we eat on our skin.

We all know that what we eat affects how our bodies look, but most of us don't realize the effects of diet on the condition of our skin. A lifestyle of excessive amounts of caffeine, alcohol, smoking and junk food will not produce beautiful skin!

For healthy, younger-looking skin, eat a balanced diet that includes significant amounts of fruits and vegetables, proteins and fiber. Avoid chemical additives and synthetic foods. A nutritionist can help you develop a good meal plan.

———◆◆◆———

TIP: Raw and natural foods produce naturally beautiful skin.

BEAUTIFUL TABLETS
Don't Forget Your Vitamins

*Certain vitamins can directly affect
the way your skin looks and acts.*

Most people equate taking vitamins with feeling good and being healthy. But vitamins have an impact on skin, as well. Here are some examples:

★ Vitamin E (vitamin E acetate) is known as an anti-aging vitamin and has a strong healing ability.

★ Vitamin A (retinyl/palmitate) is necessary for producing new cells and can be depleted by stress.

★ Vitamin C (ascorbic acid) can build collagen and elastin, which strengthen the skin. Caffeine and alcohol can deplete this vitamin.

★ Vitamin B is known as an anti-stress vitamin, and stress can greatly affect skin condition. Smoking and alcohol can deplete this vitamin.

Consult an expert to design a vitamin program just for you.

TIP: Look for skin-care products that contain vitamins that are good for your skin.

BEAUTIFUL CLEANSING
Washing Frequently and Fully

The first step of a skin-care program is the right cleanser.

Always look for natural products. Choose one that has little or no fragrance, which can be irritating to the skin, and that does not contain harsh chemicals such as soaps and detergents.

And remember, never go to bed without cleansing your face. Makeup and the impurities that the skin can attract in the course of a day can penetrate and clog the pores if not removed daily!

TIP: Never cleanse with soaps or detergents.

BEAUTIFUL NORMALIZING
Always Tone after Cleansing

After cleansing your skin, bring it back to its normal balance.

Products used to restore balance are commonly referred to as toners, normalizers or astringents. They can make a dramatic difference in the tone and texture of your skin.

When selecting a product with which to balance your skin, look for natural products that do not contain alcohol, which will strip the skin of its natural moisture balance. Also, choose products that have little or no fragrance. Aloe vera is very effective in cellular renewal.

———————

TIP: After cleansing, bring your skin into balance with a toner or normalizer.

BEAUTIFUL MOISTURE

Preventing Your Face from Drying Out

*Moisturizers protect skin from the environment
and allow smoother application of other products.*

After cleansing and toning, the third daily step in a healthy skin-care regime is to moisturize with a product that will penetrate the skin. Products that do not penetrate can clog pores and cause blemishes.

Choose a natural product that does not contain mineral oil. Apply moisturizer while your face is still damp from toning so it will penetrate faster and be more effective.

———◦◦◦◦———

TIP: Apply moisturizer immediately after toning to assure penetration.

BEAUTIFUL PEEPERS

Protecting Your Eye Area

The skin around the eyes is a very delicate area that requires special care.

It's also the place where the first signs of aging appear. Since the density of the skin around the eyes is much different from the rest of your facial skin, do not use a facial moisturizer in the eye area.

Instead, buy one of the wide variety of creams, gels and oils that are designed specifically for daily use around the eyes. Apply it to the outside edges of the lid (where you would line the lids) to keep this area from wrinkling, as well.

———◦◦◦———

TIP: Always use a moisturizer designed for the area around your eyes.

BEAUTIFUL SOMNOLENCE
Sleeping to Rest and Dream

Quality sleep time can directly affect the way we look.

Puffy eyes and dark circles are usually the result of lack of sleep. However, the position you sleep in can also affect how you look. If you sleep on your stomach or your side with your face pressed against the pillow, you will wake up with lines that can one day become more permanent.

Always try to get a good night's sleep. And train yourself to sleep on your back. Try using a chiropractic pillow, which will give proper support to your neck.

———◦◦◦◦———

TIP: Sleep on your back to avoid facial wrinkles.

BEAUTIFUL CLOWNING
Giving Yourself a Great Facial Workout

Regular exercise is important to your face.

Just as exercises keep your body fit, there are various exercises designed to stretch and develop the muscles in the skin, allowing the skin to remain firm and toned. Consult one of the many wonderful books available that can help you develop a facial exercise or "isometric" program. Doing them regularly can make a dramatic change in the tone of your facial muscles.

Moisturize the skin before doing facial exercises to increase elasticity.

TIP: Frequent facial isometrics can reduce wrinkles.

BEAUTIFUL COLOR WHEEL
Creating a Perfect Canvas

Create a beautiful base for the perfect application of makeup.

Just as painters are selective when choosing the canvas for their paintings, you must be selective when purchasing the proper foundation to give you flawless skin. Selecting a foundation is much like choosing the right moisturizer. Look for one that contains ingredients that are beneficial for healthy skin and that does not contain mineral oil.

To ensure an excellent blend, always choose the color in proper lighting. Test a small amount of foundation on your jawbone; match the skin on your neck.

———— ⋙∘⋘ ————

TIP: Proper foundation selection is key.

BEAUTIFUL HIDEOUT
Covering the Flaws

To hide imperfections in your skin tone, choose a concealer that is the right consistency for your skin.

Look for products that apply evenly and that compliment your skin tone. Never compromise. Take time in making this important decision. Application of a concealer should be made to the dark areas under the eye, around the nose, on the chin, at the top of the forehead and just under the brow bone to lighten up the eye area.

———◦◦◦◦◦———

TIP: Make sure you choose a concealer with the right consistency.

BEAUTIFUL BROWS
Framing the Eyes

The design of the brow is very important to the overall look of an eye.

To determine where the arch of the brow should occur, take a pencil and, while looking in a mirror, hold it in front of your eye. Line it up with the outer edge of your iris. The arch of your brow should be where the pencil crosses it.

———≍≎≍———

TIP: Attend to your brows regularly; wax or tweeze them to maintain their shape.

BEAUTIFUL OUTLINES
Enhancing the Eyes

Eye shadow should compliment the beauty of your eyes.

Poorly applied eye shadow can ruin an entire look. The key to applying beautiful eye shadow is to carefully blend it with an eye shadow brush and to choose colors in natural tones, browns and beiges preferably. Apply a powder foundation to the eyelids before applying shadow to make shadow easier to blend and less likely to fade away.

———⟨∞⟩———

TIP: Stay away from bold or bright eye shadow colors.

BEAUTIFUL SMUDGES

Defining the Eyes

*Eyeliner gives shape and definition to the eyes
and can make eyelashes look longer.*

Try using eye shadow applied with a thin brush as a liner for the upper lash line. Stay as close to the lash base as possible and start at the outer edge. Line only three-quarters of the eye to keep the eye more open-looking. If you choose to line under the longer lashes, choose a color that would create a smoky look, such as gray or brown.

TIP: Create more of a shadow than a line when defining the eyes.

BEAUTIFUL LASHES
Opening Your Eyes

***Use an eyelash curler to "open" your eyes
and create thicker, longer-looking lashes.***

Then apply mascara to the tips of the lashes first. Repeat application starting at the base. If you don't need a waterproof mascara, don't buy one. The chemicals that give them their staying power are not good for your lashes.

TIP: Fresh mascara creates a fresh look. Throw away and replace mascara every two to three months!

BEAUTIFUL BLUSH
Creating a Glow

*Apply blush to your cheeks to add
a natural glow to your face.*

Always apply a powder blush to a powdered face. If you apply blush directly to a clean face, your blush may become blotchy. Use a deeper tone under your cheekbones and brush it toward the ear and the hairline. Choose a softer tone on your cheeks above the bone and brush it toward the hairline, blending the two tones as they meet.

—————◦◊◦—————

TIP: Always follow blush application with loose powder to ensure proper blending.

BEAUTIFUL PUCKER
Perfecting Your Lips

Your look is not complete without perfect lips.

Lining your lips with a lip pencil is very important in creating the proper shape. You can also make lips appear to be larger or smaller with the proper line. After lining, fill in lips using a lip brush for better application and more control. Select a color that matches the liner. Remember to blot your lipstick and any remaining excess.

———◦◦◦———

TIP: Lipstick will have more staying power if you first apply foundation and powder to your lips.

BEAUTIFUL FINALE
Completing the Look

*After applying your makeup, brush
dusting powder lightly over your entire face.*

Use a large, soft brush, which will give you a natural, finishing touch. Use only quality makeup brushes, and wash them frequently to avoid a buildup of color.

———⊰∘⊱———

TIP: Choosing the right tools for makeup and selecting the right makeup are equally important.

BEAUTIFUL WISDOM
Updating with Age

Adapt your makeup to your age, style and lifestyle.

You can't wear the same makeup you wore as a teenager when you're in your fifties and sixties. Every ten years, refocus on the best makeup tips for your age. Consult a makeup artist who is not representing a specific product line; he or she will have a different motive in mind.

———◈◈◈———

TIP: Consult a makeup artist to keep up to date with current fashion and beauty trends.

BEAUTIFUL CONTRAST
Coloring to Compliment

When searching for the right makeup,
keep quality in mind.

Find the proper colors for your skin tone. Choosing a blush that is warmer in color, such as peach or coral, when your skin tone is cooler would cause a noticeable contrast. A rose or pink color would create a more consistent look. Consult with a makeup expert and explore the possibilities of custom blending.

———◦◦◦◦———

TIP: Ask a makeup professional about custom-blended colors.

BEAUTIFUL BALANCE

Take Care of Yourself

Millions long for immortality, but do not know what to do with themselves on a Sunday afternoon.

Post these "handle with care" instructions where you will see them daily—to be beautifully good to yourself first, so your beauty can shine out:

★ Simplify. Do important tasks in prime time, sort out those not worth doing, savor each task.

★ Listen to your needs. Remember what makes you happy, healthy and productive.

★ Answer your own needs. Unless you take care of yourself, you diminish what you have to offer others.

★ Know your limits. Then you can be your best without pressure.

★ Trust your feelings. They're yours, even if they differ from what you think you should be feeling.

★ Believe in yourself. Know that your beauty is shining, from the inside out, every moment, every day.

———◦◦◦———

TIP: What you practice projecting you *are* projecting and you become.

Be Now Who You Want to Be

The subconscious can't take a joke.

You will become what you dream to be by acting as if you are that person already. Give yourself constant reminders of the new you by posting positive affirmations in all parts of your life, from your makeup drawer to your laundry door to your car dashboard and your alarm clock face. See them. Say them. Find a friend for mutual reinforcement. Develop your own.

★ I am beautiful, from the inside out, as I live love.
★ I enter each situation with the gift of bringing out others' best sides.
★ I reap what I sow.
★ I always prove myself right.
★ I am all I need because I am what I desire.
★ Quieting the chattering mind promotes directed action.
★ I forgive all who have offended me; not for them, but for myself.
★ To receive more, I am willing to give more.
★ I spend on others with the consciousness of giving love.

TIP: Believe that you are giving beauty, from the inside out, into the world each moment.

About the Authors

Kare Anderson is an Emmy award-winning former TV, radio and newspaper reporter, former corporate division director, and author who speaks internationally on persuasive communication. She lives in Sausalito, California.

Kay Casperson is the founder and president of Look International, an international model and talent agency, and Pure Basics skin and hair care company which are experiencing explosive growth. She lives in Minneapolis.

The authors are available as conference speakers. Please contact MasterMedia's Speakers' Bureau for availability and fee arrangements. **Call Tony Colao at (800) 453-2887 or (908) 359-1612 or fax (908) 359-1647.**

MasterMedia Limited

To order copies of *Beauty Inside Out* ($8.95), send a check for the price of each book ordered plus $2 postage and handling for the first book and $1 for each additional copy to:

MasterMedia Limited
17 East 89th Street
New York, NY 10128
(212) 546-7650
(800) 334-8232
(212) 546-7638 (fax)
(Please use MasterCard or VISA on phone orders)

An Invitation

If you found this book helpful and want to receive a MasterMedia book catalog or a newsletter that contains a list of MasterMedia's inspirational books that carry the Heritage Imprint, write or fax to the above address or phone number.

MasterMedia is the only company to combine publishing with a full-service speakers' bureau.

MasterMedia books and speakers cover today's important issues—from family values to health topics and business ethics.

For information and a complete list of speakers, call (800) 453-2887 or fax (908) 359-1647.

Special Offer to *Beauty Inside Out* Readers

Each *Beauty Inside Out* reader can receive a free gift from co-author Kay Casperson's skin- and hair-care line, Pure Basics. Just fill out and fax or mail this page to:

> **Kay Casperson**
> **Look International**
> **7407 Wayzata Blvd.**
> **St. Louis Park, MN 55426**
> **(612) 595-8615 (fax)**

___ Yes, I am committed to living the theme of *Beauty Inside Out* and becoming positively unforgettable. Please send my free gift from Pure Basics.

NAME _____

STREET ADDRESS _____

CITY _____

STATE _____

ZIP CODE _____

DAYTIME PHONE _____

EVENING PHONE _____

Four Special Offers on Kare Anderson's
Three New Books to Learn to "Say It Better"

Offer #1
Order all three of Kare Anderson's new condensed pocket books (available May 1996) and get a free copy of T. Scott Gross's *Pocket POS* or deduct 20% from the cover prices

___ send *Pocket POS* ($32.85 enclosed)

___ deduct 20% ($27.48 enclosed)

Offer #2
Order two sets of Kare Anderson's three-book collection (great gifts for friends, colleagues, corporate recognition programs and conference mementos) and receive her hot tips: "26 Ways to Attract More Customers and More Per-Customer Spending Through 800 Numbers, Other Phone Services and FaxBacks."

___ send two sets and the tips ($67.50 enclosed)

Offer #3
Bring Kare Anderson to speak at your meeting and receive twenty free, autographed copies of her books (you choose the mix) to sell or give away at your meeting (indicate the quantity you want of each):

___ *Pocket Beauty Inside Out*

___ *Pocket Cross-Promotional Marketing*

___ *Pocket Persuasion & Negotiation Tips*

Offer #4
Recommend Kare Anderson to an organization for which her message would be appropriate and, for making this referral, receive a free copy of one of her books (choose one below):

___ *Pocket Beauty Inside Out*

___ *Pocket Cross-Promotional Marketing*

___ *Pocket Persuasion & Negotiation Tips*

Yes, I want to take advantage of one of these offers:

___ #1 (check for $32.85 or $27.48 enclosed)

___ #2 (check for $65.70 enclosed)

___ #3 (Kare Anderson to speak at your meeting)

___ #4 (referral)

Prices include $2 per book for mailing, handling and tax.
Please make checks payable to MasterMedia Limited.

Mail or fax responses (see following page) to offers #1 and #2 to:
MasterMedia Limited
17 East 89th Street
New York, NY 10128
(800) 334-8232
(212) 546-7650
(212) 546-7638 (fax)
(Please use MasterCard or
VISA on fax orders)

Mail or fax responses to offers #3 and #4 to:
Tony Colao
MasterMedia Limited
17 East 89th Street
New York, NY 10128
(800) 453-2887
(908) 359-1612
(908) 359-1647 (fax)

YOUR NAME _____

DAYTIME PHONE _____

ORGANIZATION _____

STREET ADDRESS _____

CITY _____

STATE _____

ZIP CODE _____

MEETING (IF ANY) AT WHICH
KARE ANDERSON'S MESSAGE
WOULD BE RELEVANT _____

DATE OF MEETING _____

NAME OF COLLEAGUE WHO HIRES SPEAKERS _____

DAYTIME PHONE _____

ORGANIZATION _____

STREET ADDRESS _____

CITY _____

STATE _____

ZIP CODE _____

KIND OF MEETING FOR WHICH COLLEAGUE
BRINGS IN OUTSIDE SPEAKERS _____

DATE OF MEETING _____

To learn about Kare Anderson's other educational products, please ask her office to send a product information sheet (check one):

___ please mail product information

___ please fax product information

NAME _____

DAYTIME PHONE _____

FAX _____

ORGANIZATION _____

STREET ADDRESS _____

CITY _____

STATE _____

ZIP CODE _____

Mail or fax responses:
The Kare Anderson Company
15 Sausalito Blvd.
Sausalito, CA 94965
(415) 331-6336
(415) 331-6661 (fax)

Or, to find out about speaking engagements, please call Tony Colao at MasterMedia's Speaker's Bureau, (800) 453-2887.

OTHER MASTERMEDIA BOOKS

To order additional copies of any MasterMedia book, send a check for the price of the book plus $2.00 postage and handling for the first book, $1.00 for each additional book to:

MasterMedia Limited
17 East 89th Street
New York, NY 10128
(212) 546-7650
(800) 334-8232
(212) 546-7638 (fax)
(Please use MasterCard or VISA on phone orders)

AGING PARENTS AND YOU: A Complete Handbook to Help You Help Your Elders Maintain a Healthy, Productive and Independent Life, by Eugenia Anderson-Ellis, is a complete guide to providing care to aging relatives. It gives practical advice and resources to adults who are helping their elders lead productive and independent lives. Revised and updated. ($9.95 paper)

BALANCING ACTS! Juggling Love, Work, Family, and Recreation, by Susan Schiffer Stautberg and Marcia L. Worthing, provides strategies to achieve a balanced life by reordering priorities and setting realistic goals. ($12.95 paper)

BEATING THE AGE GAME: Redefining Retirement, by Jack and Phoebe Ballard, debunks the myth that retirement means sitting out the rest of the game. The years between 55 and 80 can be your best, say the authors, who provide ample examples of people successfully using retirement to reinvent their lives. ($12.95 paper)

THE BIG APPLE BUSINESS AND PLEASURE GUIDE: 501 Ways to Work Smarter, Play Harder, and Live Better in New York City, by Muriel Siebert and Susan Kleinman, offers visitors and New Yorkers alike advice on how to do business in the city and enjoy its attractions. ($9.95 paper)

BREATHING SPACE: Living and Working at a Comfortable Pace in a Sped-Up Society, by Jeff Davidson, helps readers to handle information and activity overload and gain greater control over their lives. ($10.95 paper)

CARVING WOOD AND STONE, by Arnold Prince, is an illustrated step-by-step handbook demonstrating all you need to hone your wood and carving skills. ($11.95 paper)

THE COLLEGE COOKBOOK II, for Students by Students, by Nancy Levicki, is a handy volume of recipes culled from college students across the U.S. ($11.95)

THE CONFIDENCE FACTOR: How Self-Esteem Can Change Your Life, by Dr. Judith Briles, is based on a nationwide survey of six thousand men and women. Briles explores why women so often feel a lack of self-confidence and have a poor opinion of themselves. She offers step-by-step advice on becoming the person you want to be. ($9.95 paper, $18.95 cloth)

CUPID, COUPLES & CONTRACTS: A Guide to Living Together, Prenuptial Agreements, and Divorce, by Lester Wallman, with Sharon McDonnell, is an insightful, consumer-oriented handbook that provides a comprehensive overview of family law, including prenuptial agreements, alimony and fathers' rights ($12.95 paper)

THE DOLLARS AND SENSE OF DIVORCE: The Financial Guide for Women, by Dr. Judith Briles, is the first book to combine the legal hurdles by planning finances before, during and after divorce. ($10.95 paper)

FINANCIAL SAVVY FOR WOMEN: A Money Book for Women of All Ages, by Dr. Judith Briles, divides a woman's monetary lifespan into six phases, discusses specific issues to be addressed at each stage and demonstrates how to create a sound money plan. ($15.00 paper)

FLIGHT PLAN FOR LIVING: The Art of Self-Encouragement, by Patrick O'Dooley, is a guide organized like a pilot's checklist, to ensure you'll by flying "clear to the top" throughout your life. ($17.95 cloth)

HOT HEALTH-CARE CAREERS, by Margaret McNally and Phyllis Schneider, offers readers what they need to know about training for and getting jobs in a rewarding field where professionals are always in demand. ($10.95 paper)

HOW TO GET WHAT YOU WANT FROM ALMOST ANYBODY, by T. Scott Gross, shows how to get great service, negotiate better prices and always get what you pay for. ($9.95 paper)

KIDS WHO MAKE A DIFFERENCE, by Joyce Roché and Marie Rodriguez, is an inspiring document on how today's toughest challenges are being met by teenagers and kids, whose courage and creativity enables them to find practical solutions! ($8.95 paper, with photos)

LEADING YOUR POSITIVELY OUTRAGEOUS SERVICE TEAM, by T. Scott Gross, forgoes theory in favor of a hands-on approach. Gross provides a step-by-step formula for developing self-managing service teams that put the customer first. ($12.95 paper)

LIFE'S THIRD ACT: Taking Control of Your Mature Years, by Patricia Burnham, Ph.D., is a perceptive handbook for everyone who recognizes that planning is the key to enjoying your mature years. ($10.95 paper, $18.95 cloth)

LIFETIME EMPLOYABILITY: How to Become Indispensable, by Carole Hyatt is both a guide through the mysteries of the business universe brought down to earth and a handbook to help you evaluate your attitudes, your skills, and your goals. Through expert advice and interviews of nearly 200 men and women whose lives have changed because their jobs or goals shifted, *Lifetime Employability* is designed to increase your staying power in today's down-sized economy. ($12.95 paper)

LISTEN TO WIN: A Guide to Effective Listening, by Curt Bechler, Ph.D., and Richard Weaver, Ph.D., is a powerful, people-oriented book that will help you learn to live with others, connect with them and get the best from them. ($18.95 cloth)

THE LIVING HEART BRAND NAME SHOPPER'S GUIDE, by Michael F. DeBakey, M.D., Antonio M. Gotto, Jr., M.D., Lynne W. Scott, M.A., R.D./L.D., and John P. Foreyt, Ph.D., lists brand-name supermarket products that are low in fat, saturated fatty acids, and cholesterol. ($12.50 paper)

THE LIVING HEART GUIDE TO EATING OUT, by Michael F. DeBakey, M.D., Antonio M. Gotto, Jr., M.D., and Lynne W. Scott, M.A., R.D./L.D., is an essential handbook for people who want to maintain a health-conscious diet when dining in all types of restaurants. ($9.95 paper)

MAKING YOUR DREAMS COME TRUE NOW!, by Marcia Wieder, introduces an easy, unique, and practical technique for defining, pursuing, and realizing your career and life interests. Filled with stories of real people and helpful exercises, plus a personal workbook. (Revised and updated. $10.95 paper)

MANAGING IT ALL: Time-Saving Ideas for Career, Family, Relationships, and Self, by Beverly Benz Treuille and Susan Schiffer Stautberg, is written for women who are juggling careers and families. More than 200 career women (ranging from a TV anchorwoman to an investment baker) were interviewed. The book contains many humorous anecdotes on saving time and improving the quality of life for self and family. ($9.95 paper)

MANAGING YOUR CHILD'S DIABETES, by Robert Wood Johnson IV, Sale Johnson, Casey Johnson, and Susan Kleinman, brings help to families trying to understand diabetes and control its effects. ($10.95 paper)

MANAGING YOUR PSORIASIS, by Nicholas J. Lowe, M.D., is an innovative manual that couples scientific research and encouraging support, with an emphasis on how patients can take charge of their health. ($10.95 paper, $17.95 cloth)

MANN FOR ALL SEASONS: Wit and Wisdom from The Washington Post's Judy Mann, shows the columnist at her best as she writes about women, families and the impact and politics of the women's revolution. ($9.95 paper, $19.95 cloth)

MEMORY: Remembering and Forgetting in Everyday Life, by Dr. Barry Gordon, explains the difference between a real memory impairment and the normal absent-mindedness that affects us all. ($25.00 cloth)

MIND YOUR OWN BUSINESS: And Keep It in the Family, by Marcy Syms, CEO of Syms Corp., is an effective guide for any organization facing the toughest step in managing a family business—making the transition to the new generation. ($12.95 paper, $18.95 cloth)

OFFICE BIOLOGY: Why Tuesday Is the Most Productive Day and Other Relevant Facts for Survival in the Workplace, by Edith Weiner and Arnold Brown, teaches how in the '90s and beyond we will be expected to work smarter, take better control of our health, adapt to advancing technology, and improve our lives in ways that are not too costly or resource-intensive. ($12.95 paper, $21.95 cloth)

ON TARGET: Enhance Your Life and Advance Your Career, by Jeri Sedlar and Rick Miners, is a neatly woven tapestry of insights on career and life issues gathered from audiences across the country. This feedback has been crystallized into a highly readable guide for exploring what you want. ($11.95 paper)

PAIN RELIEF: How to Say No to Acute, Chronic, and Cancer Pain!, by Dr. Jane Cowles, offers a step-by-step plan for assessing pain and communicating it to your doctor, and explains the importance of having a pain plan before undergoing any medical or surgical treatment; includes "The Pain Patient's Bill of Rights," and a reusable pain assessment chart. ($14.95 paper, 22.95 cloth)

POSITIVELY OUTRAGEOUS SERVICE: New and Easy Ways to Win Customers for Life, by T. Scott Gross, identifies what '90s consumers really want and how business can develop effective marketing strategies to answer those needs. ($14.95 paper)

THE PREGNANCY AND MOTHERHOOD DIARY: Planning the First Year of Your Second Career, by Susan Schiffer Stautberg, is the first and only undated appointment diary that shows how to manage pregnancy and career. ($12.95, spiral bound)

ROSEY GRIER'S ALL-AMERICAN HEROES: Multicultural Success Stories, by Roosevelt "Rosey" Grier, is a candid collection of profiles of prominent African-

Americans, Latins, Asians and Native Americans who reveal how they achieved public acclaim and personal success. ($9.95 paper, with photos)

A SEAT AT THE TABLE: An Insider's Guide for America's New Women Leaders, by Patricia Harrison. A must-read guide that offers practical advice for women who want to serve on boards of directors, play key roles in politics and community affairs or become policy makers in public or private sectors. ($19.95 cloth)

SELLING YOURSELF: Be the Competent, Confident Person You Really Are!, by Kathy Thebo, Joyce Newman and Diana Lynn. The ability to express yourself effectively and to project a confident image is essential in today's fast-paced world where professional and personal lines frequently cross. ($12.95 paper)

SHOCKWAVES. The Global Impact of Sexual Harassment, by Susan L. Webb, examines the problem of sexual harassment today in every kind of workplace around the world. Well-researched, this manual provides the most recent information available, including legal changes in progress. ($11.95 paper, $19.95 cloth)

SOMEONE ELSE'S SON, by Alan Winter, explores the parent-child bond in a contemporary novel of lost identities, family secrets and relationships gone awry. Eighteen years after bringing their first son home from the hospital, Tish and Brad Hunter discover they are not his biological parents. ($18.95 cloth)

STEP FORWARD: Sexual Harassment in the Workplace, What You Need to Know, by Susan L. Webb, presents the facts for identifying the tell-tale signs of sexual harassment on the job, and how to deal with it. ($9.95 paper)

THE STEPPARENT CHALLENGE: A Primer for Making it Work, by Stephen Williams, Ph.D., offers insight into the many aspects of step relationships—from financial issues to lifestyle changes to differences in race and or religion that affect the whole family. ($13.95 paper)

STRAIGHT TALK ON WOMEN'S HEALTH: How to Get the Health Care You Deserve, by Janice Teal, Ph.D., and Phyllis Schneider, is destined to become a health-care "bible." Devoid of confusing medical jargon, it offers a wealth of resources, including contact lists of health lines and women's medical centers. ($14.95 paper)

WHEN THE WRONG THING IS RIGHT: How to Overcome Conventional Wisdom, Popular Opinion and All the Lies Your Parents Told You, by Sylvia Bigelson, Ed.S., and Virginia McCullough, addresses issues such as marriage, relationships, parents and siblings, divorce, sex, money and careers, and encourages readers to break free from the pressures of common wisdom and to trust their own choices. ($9.95 paper)